YOU ARE THE LIGHT

---

21 Days To Your New Life Habit

by Hana

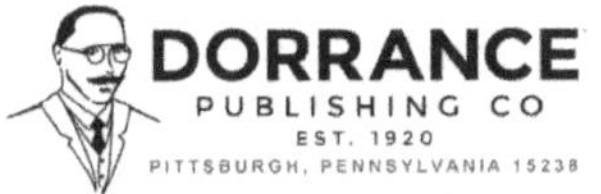

Dorrance Publishing Co
585 Alpha Drive
Pittsburgh, PA 15238
Visit our website at *www.dorrancebookstore.com*

ISBN: 979-8-88729-261-8
eISBN: 979-8-88729-761-3

YOU ARE THE LIGHT

21 Days To Your New Life Habit

Dedication

This is dedicated to anyone at the bookstore seeing all those big self help books, feeling overwhelmed already. Start here, this book is for anyone who's ever felt like the Horse in the Never Ending Story.

To my children Gavin & Lyv, never forget you help keep my lantern on full glow and you too have that ability for yourself. Never lose sight throughout this journey that you are enough. I love you.

To everyone who's filled my heart even if just for a moment. You've helped my life feel lived and for that I'm forever grateful.

Hana

Introduction

I'll keep this short and sweet, I can't take too long to capture your attention. Or, re-alistically, to have you commit to this quick journey that can change you for a lifetime.

We are at the proverbial fork in the road. Our beacon is on low, and the tunnel is dark. I won't lie to you and tell you some-one is at the end of the tunnel waving the white flag. What I will tell you is what you remember at the earliest, happiest childhood memory. That you, YES YOU, are the light.

Day 1 – Breathe

Throughout the next 21 days, I need you to practice breathing.

Your breath will steady you. It's our inner navigation system, our soul compass. It will bring you back to you.

Simple: Today, and every day there-after, commit to 6 deep breaths and say the word "reset" in your head each time.

Do this before you get out of bed each morning, and any time your breath seems to escape you.

Daily Journey: 6 Breaths – Inhale (say reset) – Exhale

Day 2 – Leave Your Shit at the Door

When you enter your workplace today, or maybe whatever appointment you may have, or social engagement, before entering, drop all of the baggage and heaviness you've been carrying in the imaginary box at the door. I promise you it's safe there, no one wants your shit, they have their own.

Release that heavy load, for a little while, and enter as your best self. Take the sun glasses off, engage the room, and smile.

(Don't forget to breathe.)

Daily Journey: Don't bring the noise with you today.

Day 3 – It's Showtime

That's the mentality. You're the lead of your life, the starring role. You can't let an understudy take your place. You're ir-replaceable. Keep that positive self-talk. Don't even joke negatively about your-self. Words cast spells; that's why they call it spelling (so it's been said).

Daily Journey: Practice positive man-tras, such as 'I am deserving,' 'Why not me?' 'My past is not my present'. To en-tice, say it out loud thrice.

Day 4 – Turn Off the News

Take a breather from all social media outlets today. Stay in a media-free bubble for the entire day. I'm talking speak, read, listen or entertain mere mention of current events.

Daily Journey: Instead, turn on home movies, flip through sentimental photo albums and find those old school agendas and yearbooks. (Weren't you awesome?)

Day 5 – Be Your Own PR

Who can market yourself better than you? Show up for yourself in some way shape or form. We are always advocating for others and that's great; don't forget that you need some of that shine on yourself.

Daily Journey: Use your social media, or any platform you choose, or maybe just tell the person next to you that you yourself in fact *rock*!

Day 6 – Dust Your Shoulders Off

No matter how much we PR ourselves we sometimes have a pesky memory or voice in our head (also known as our ego) that tries hard to keep us in a prior pattern because the ego only knows what's already happened and cannot direct you past yesterday.

Daily Journey: Firstly, look up online what exactly your ego is. You've been taught incorrectly. Afterwards, thank your ego for always trying to protect you and keep you safe. Then dust your shoulders off and recite the mantras from Day 3.

Day 7 – Check Up from the Neck Up

Wow, one week. What worked? What didn't? Why didn't it?

What's your recipe for improvement? How will you start incorporating all 6 days into practice effective today, Day 7!

Daily Journey: Impact yourself and take tips from all of the days so far and start making it a habit.

Day 8 – Hold a Meeting

Now is the time for an accountability check. Where do you take shortcuts on your mental and physical health? Come prepared to your self-evaluation with your recipe for improvement from day 6. Took a shortcut and didn't do it? Well get to work, we'll wait.

Daily Journey: Set those benchmarks for improvement from the last week and be ready to implement.

Day 9 – Insert Music

Put your playlist on shuffle. Click the next song. What message is in those song lyrics you're listening to? How do they resonate?

Daily Journey: Journal about the song and what feelings it invoked in you. How has music healed you through the years? How can you incorporate more music into your life?

Day 10 – Ground Yourself

Reconnect to the earth. It's one of nature's hidden therapies. The electrical charge straight from the Earth has been known to have positive effects on our own bodies. There is nothing like walking barefoot outside or hugging a tree. There are so many benefits from getting outdoors and being one with nature.

Daily Journey: Find a safe place and spend 20 minutes practicing quiet grounding.

Day 11 – Say NO

Today is a great day to say "NO". Two letters, so tough to say sometimes. Why is that pesky small word so painful to speak? Well, it means we show up as our authentic self and put ourselves first.

Daily Journey: Say "NO" today. At the very least tell someone you'll think about it to give yourself time to build courage, then say "No".

Day 12 – Reach Out

Who's on your mind today? Who is always near your mind's eye? Sometimes we have people, whether here with us or departed, that hold space in our thoughts.

Daily Journey: Reach out to them today. Whether it's through a phone call, email or even just journaling a letter, let's express how much they mean to us.

Day 13 – Dance

Physical activity is crucial to this new you. Sometimes being told to go to the gym for an hour or go for a run can ripple a lot of lethargic thoughts into your head. Using a song that ramps you up or makes you sway is all you need to change the energy within.

Daily Journey: Take 5 minutes minimum and get physical.

Increase as YOU see fit.

Day 14 – How's That Breath Work and Grounding Going?

Are we committed to the shift you're feeling? Are you channeling the last 14 days and uniting them in the melody called your life? This last week was tough to stay consistent maybe. Did you? Don't get down, get even. Keep it up. This upcoming week is where it stops being work to care about yourself and the week in which you start to glow.

Daily Journey: Ask the universe to turn up your inner lantern.

Day 15 – Notice How You Carry Yourself

How you carry yourself is an integral part of this journey. When we are sad or fearful, our bodies close up, we don't stand tall and we want to withdraw. Focusing on how you carry yourself will shift your entire mindset from "I'm fearful" to "I'm fearless."

Daily Journey: Notice how you carry yourself and make a constant effort today to stand tall. Shoulders back, chin up and smile.

Day 16 – Look at the Moon

The wondrous moon. Like you, it's perfect at every phase, dark to full. Embrace all of your phases and team up with the moon to mirror that mindset.

Daily Journey: Go look up at the moon tonight and star gaze.

Don't forget to make a wish.

Day 17 – Read an Article on Oneness

We read so much, but what exactly are we reading? What are we in taking into our system and allowing to be a part of our thoughts and knowledge? Take some time to learn about oneness, it's something not mainstream, but collectively the most inspiring. We are all one, with each other, and the inner work we are doing will lead us to this mindset.

Daily Journey: Read up and learn about oneness.

Day 18 – Book That Self Care

We need to make certain that this avatar of a human vessel we are in is too getting the self care it deserves. It will make your soul glow and your vision flow.

Daily Journey: Book that massage, Reiki session, spa day you always put off. You deserve it!

Day 19 – Feel the Burn

You are starting to realize that you are waking up feeling warm and more whole than you have in so long. You radiate the energy of a beautiful fire in the dark nights of winter. How magical.

Daily Journey: Sit still with yourself for a few moments and just feel the warmth of your glow. Smile and drink it in.

Day 20 – Never Settle

No one gets to dictate who you are and what you can achieve. If a door closes there is always a window of new opportunity.

Remember 'Why not you?'

Daily Journey: Break open the constraints of your mindset. Start reaching further towards your inner goals that you truly want to achieve.

Day 21 – YOU ARE THE LIGHT

Wow, you made it. Here we are, top of the peak, air's good in our lungs; we are breathing it in and the inner lantern is full glow.

These days filled you with everything you already knew. That you, yes you, are the light.

Remember at the top of the peak means more mountains to go down and climb. But with the inner knowing, yes knowing, that you are capable, you may enjoy the hike.

Life Journey: Live these days for a life-time.